Crohn's disease and my journey to better health

Foreword

My Journey with Crohn's disease, the healing process and trials and tribulations

Why this book? I want to share with you everything I've been through in the last 20 years or so dealing with my Crohn's disease and my journey to better health and healing. I have tried countless of diets, supplements and read books and done hundreds of hours of research on Crohn's disease and autoimmune diseases in general. This book is a consolidated version of everything I've learned and tried myself. I hope this book will bring you hope if you have been just diagnosed with this disease or you have had the disease for a long time and are looking for something, anything to help you. I also wrote this book to help you if you are a parent or a caregiver wanting to help your loved one manage Crohn's, colitis, IBS or an autoimmune disease. I've spent almost half of my life time dealing with Crohn's disease but the last several years I've been on the healing journey. Today I'm medication and mostly symptom free and have been in remission for several years now. Please note that I'm not a medical doctor and this book is not intended to cure, prevent or treat any diseases. I'm purely sharing my journey in hopes of helping others. I'm a certified Health Coach through American Association of Drugless Practitioners and a certified essential oil coach. I want to share everything I've learned over several years by doing my research, trying different things myself through trial and error as well as everything I've learned through my training of becoming a certified Health coach through American Association of Drugless practitioners. I'm passionate about helping others and sharing this information because my healing process has made such a difference in my life and in the quality of my life. I want to help others looking for ways to manage their disease naturally by sharing everything I know so that you can take charge of your own health as well. Please note the information and products mentioned in this book have not been evaluated by the Food and Drug Administration and are not intended to diagnose, treat, cure or prevent any disease. I'm not a medical doctor and this book is not intended for medical advice. Always check with your doctor if you have existing medical concerns.

Table of Contents

by Reija Eden - AADP Health Coach & Certified Essential Oil Coach...1

Foreword..1

My Journey with Crohn's disease, the healing process and trials and tribulations 1

My Crohn's Diagnosis..5

My 20s & 30s...7

Pregnancies & Loss 10

My Quest for Healing 12

Paleo diet & My Healing Process............................15

Food Sensitivity Testing 16

Root Causes and Modern Medicine 18

Leaky Gut and skin issues 20

What is a leaky gut? 21

How do you heal a leaky gut? 22

What finally put me on the path of healing & My Diet.......................23

What's a Paleo Diet? 25

What can you do to support your body with starting a healing process?...26

How to Get Started With Healthier Diet................29

Sample daily meals..31

My Diet today...34

My sample daily diet...37

Emotional Health 40

Remove Toxins 41

Resources 42

Crohn's disease
and my journey to better health naturally

Reija Eden - AADP Certified Health Coach & Essential Oil Coach

My Crohn's Diagnosis

It was 1996, my senior year in high school and I was feeling horrible day and day out. I was in and out of hospitals because I had high fevers that would only go away with rounds and rounds of antibiotics. The doctors could not figure out what was wrong with me. Every time I was on a course of antibiotics, I ended up feeling better but shortly after the course ended, my pains and horrible feeling came back along with high fevers. I was scheduled for a laparoscopy after several ultrasounds couldn't find anything specific. My blood showed high markers for infection but the doctors were not able to figure out where the inflammation was. The initial thought was that I had some female reproductive issues which turned out to be false. During the laparoscopy procedure it was discovered that I had extreme inflammation in my testiness that resulted in emergency surgery. The doctors performed the surgery and took a biopsy to determine what the cause of the inflammation was.

I was diagnosed with Crohn's disease and in my case Crohn's was found to be in the most common spot, between the large and the small intestines. They had to remove parts of both intestines because the inflammation was so severe. I remember waking up from the procedure, not knowing what just had taken place with a row of stitches on my stomach. I felt absolutely horrible and the pain from the surgery was even worse. A doctor from the hospital came to do his rounds and stopped by my bed, telling me I had Crohn's disease. I had no idea what that meant. I didn't know if it was something that I was going to die from or if it was something I was just going to have to learn to live with. I was in utter shock and didn't know if I should be happy or sad. I was relieved to finally know what was wrong with me because the years prior I had felt so horrible but the future was so unknown that I didn't really know what to think. I couldn't eat anything the days after the surgery so I lost a significant amount of weight. I finally was released to go home but I had to stay on liquid and soft food diet for a couple of days. I remember being absolutely miserable and in so much pain from my surgery.

I started the healing process slowly and the process of accepting my disease and diagnosis. I had days of "why me" but I just decided to concentrate on the everyday life and keeping myself busy. Going out to places with friends was difficult because I always needed to know where the bathroom was. Every time I ate, I had to find the bathroom. Pretty much everything I ate went straight through me. I ended up being put on medication, Asacol, to manage my disease. I was told there is no evidence if it really helps or not but it was the most common way to treat the disease at that time. I was also not given any guidance on a diet or what foods to eat and what to avoid. I just ate the foods I had eaten before not knowing that diets can affect Crohn's greatly. It wasn't until later, several years into the disease that I learned about the importance of diets. I was on the medication for several years and had both good and bad days on and off and it seemed like there was no rime a reason why some days I felt better than other days.

My 20s & 30s

I spent my 20s and 30s dealing with the disease and the symptoms the best I could. I quickly learned I couldn't eat high fiber foods or I would get major stomach pains and other troubles. I avoided healthy foods because fiber seemed to give me trouble. I ate pretty bland diet. I was afraid to eat salads because the few times I did, my stomach pains would come back or I would have what I called a "blockage" where the food doesn't seem to get digested at all. I would eat something and my stomach would completely swell up and I would end up throwing up because my stomach couldn't handle the food. I would have several cramps and nausea for 12-24 hours after the episode.

I never knew what would bring it on because it seemed to be so random. Some days I could eat food regularly and the next time I ate the same food, I would end up with the "blockage" type of episode being sick for a day or so.

Blockage

My first pregnancy in 2000 ended up actually being the first time I felt really good with my disease. I ate foods with no problems and I felt overall really good. Pregnancy has the tendency to put the disease in remission. I was really enjoying every day while being pregnant. It wasn't until after the pregnancy that my symptoms returned. My "blockage" type of episodes returned where I would eat a meal that I had eaten several times before and now all of a sudden it would give me a problem. I would throw up and be in severe pain and it would take about 24-48 hours to clear.

If you have a Crohn's disease and you are reading this I'm sure you can relate. It's the feeling of the food you just ate, not going anywhere. My stomach would start to hurt as the hours went by and finally several hours later I would throw it all up. My stomach would be tender and really sore for 24-48 hours after and many times I couldn't get out of bed because of the weakness from throwing up and the pain in my stomach. I used to say that the pains were worse than any labor pains. My stomach would go in waves and the pain would come and go. Every time this happened, my husband had to take care of me and our children because I was unable to.

I don't know the scientific reasoning or name for what I call the blockage and not sure if every person with Crohn's has it but all I knew was that I needed to avoid it at all costs. It made me so miserable and unable to do anything for several days usually. Also my stomach would be very tender to touch for a couple of days.

For many years, I continued to deal with the disease the best I could and tried to avoid any high fiber foods, thinking they were the problem for me even though sometimes these episodes would come out of nowhere even when eating foods that normally seemed to agree with me.

Pregnancies & Loss

In 2005, I ended up getting pregnant second time and my husband and I were so excited. Unfortunately the pregnancy ended as a late term loss. I had bleeding on and off after 12 weeks and finally my body rejected the pregnancy and I had to drive to the hospital bleeding profusely. The pregnancy loss was very difficult to get through and it didn't help with my Crohn's disease which seemed to be affected badly by stress and negative emotions. I had a flare that eventually calmed down on its own but the never ending bathroom trips were difficult to deal with.

I ended up getting pregnant again the following year but this time my disease didn't go into remission. Actually just the opposite, it seemed like my disease went on overdrive and I was put on Asacol to manage my symptoms. I had symptoms on and off throughout the pregnancy even with Asacol. I was told that taking Asacol during pregnancy was safe. Looking I wish I had refused the medication and just dealt with the disease but I trusted my doctor. Our daughter was born with asymmetrical crying faces which meant the muscles on one side of the mouth didn't work properly and I can't help but think that the medication was the reason. I didn't take Asacol with my other pregnancies and my other children didn't have any medical problems at birth.

It wasn't until after the pregnancy that my Crohn's symptoms got even worse. Every time I would sit to breastfeed my baby, I would have to go to the bathroom. It was extremely difficult to manage a newborn, a 5 year old and my disease at the same time. I just kept going and eventually returned back to work getting by day by day.

Everything really is a blur from that moment on other than I just ended up having to deal with my disease while going in full swing and having to go to work and deal with going to the bathroom several times a day, even at work. Asacol didn't seem to make much of a difference but I wasn't that keen on seeing my gastroenterologist knowing that there really is no cure for Crohn's and I figured it wouldn't change things much anyhow. I also didn't want to take medication but took Asacol reluctantly.

I ended up having a colonoscopy which revealed that my Crohn's had return to the same spot, between the large and small intestines. My gastroenterologist "opened" the area up during the colonoscopy so that it wouldn't close up again. After the colonoscopy I ended up having to go to the bathroom several times a day after every time I ate. My intestines seemed to have gone on overdrive again from the procedure.

I don't know how but I just kept plugging along and dealing with the daily symptoms of having to go to the bathroom several times a day and dealing with the stomach pains. The stomach pains were sometimes so bad, they almost took my breath away and all I could do was sit curled up on a couch.

Fast forward another couple of years, I did end up having another colonoscopy that revealed Crohn's being active still but luckily I didn't have as much narrowing. My prescription for Asacol ran out and I didn't go back to renew it. I had this feeling that there had to be a better way and I was determined to find it. I also wasn't convinced that the medication was really helping me that much anyway because with or without the medicine I still had symptoms.

My Quest for Healing

I was desperately for help. I was so tired of dealing with the disease and once again I was sitting on the couch trying to figure out what could help me. My stomach was going in waves and it was beyond painful. I was so miserable and in so much pain I couldn't even talk. I knew medicines weren't the answer since I had had symptoms even on the medication and I wasn't feeling any better. I also wasn't interested in taking medication that suppresses your immune system because of the potential other problems that it can cause. I thought there had to be a reason why my body was reacting this way and just masking the problem with medicines isn't what I was looking for. I wanted to get to the root of why my body was broken.

I was at a point where I was determined to find something, anything to help me. I had read several books on diets and autoimmune diseases and I had tried several different diets with various successes. I had read books on Crohn's and diets and had tried different things. Nothing seemed to really make a difference. I knew I couldn't go on like this for the rest of my life. I was so tired of the pains, always feeling so tired and having to go to the bathroom all the time.

I scoured the internet once again as I had done so many times prior and landed on Celiac forum. Someone had mentioned using Enterolabs for testing for food sensitivities. After reading that a light bulb went on in my head and I started to think that maybe I had some food sensitivities as well that could be adding to my Crohn's symptoms. I ordered a test through Enterolabs, which was a stool test, and anxiously waited for the results. I liked the idea of a stool test because I knew it had less room for error than a blood test. The results came back positive to gluten, milk, egg and soy intolerance. I immediately sprang into action and removed all of them from my diet. I did a strict elimination diet. I did a lot of research on diets and elimination diets and just decided to remove gluten, milk, egg and soy and also all possible grains. It was very difficult at first because there was not much I could eat or at least I didn't know what I could eat. I also started taking coconut oil supplements because I was not keen on eating coconut oil and didn't care for the taste. I had done research online and found that many people with Crohn's, found relief with consuming coconut oil. Coconut oil is considered having anti-viral and anti-bacterial properties. I also took evening primrose, black seed oil supplements and fish oil supplements after doing research and learning that the oils are great with their anti-inflammatory properties. I also started researching raw foods and raw food diets. I started making some raw food desserts etc. I also started to make my own almond milk by purchasing almonds in the store, soaking them overnight and making my almond milk the following day. Slowly but surely I started to feel better. It was a slow process of several months. From the moment I went on the elimination diet to the time I started to feel great daily was about 3 months. Going on the elimination diet was not an instant fix for me but I was determined to keep going and see how my body was going to react. When I started to feel better, I got even more encouraged to keep going. It was amazing that I was able to all of sudden eat higher fiber foods when I had avoided them the last several years. Later on after doing research I learned that if you have gluten intolerance, it can take 30-days or more to fully get it out of your system. If you have tried going gluten free before and you didn't feel much different, I encourage you to try again and commit to going 100% gluten free for a long period of time.

Paleo diet & My Healing Process

After about 3 months on the elimination diet, I started to feel like a whole new person. I kept going on the diet and finally stumbled across Paleo diet. I switched to Paleo diet and also discovered blogs such as Against All Grain, Elena's Pantry and Mark's Daily Apple. I was so happy to finally find a diet that I felt like I could eat a lot of foods on and they were tasty foods.

I had an appointment with my gastroenterologist and showed him the results of my stool test from Enterolabs that showed my food sensitivities. I also tried to telling him about the Paleo diet I was on and how much better I was feeling finally. Unfortunately he was not open to hearing any of it. This made me so upset because what I was sharing with the doctor could potentially help others with Crohn's. Everybody's body is different and reacts differently to foods so what was working for me might not work for everyone but it's still worth the try. I was disappointed that a gastroenterologist was not interested in hearing what I had to say that could potentially help other patients. People can have different food sensitives, different from mine. I was so upset that my doctor wouldn't even want to listen to what I was doing that was helping me.

Food Sensitivity Testing

Is everyone who has Crohn's going to have the same sensitivities as me? No, of course not, but getting testing done to see if there are any underlying food sensitives should be the first thing with anyone suffering from inflammatory bowel diseases or autoimmune diseases. By removing allergens from your diet and getting testing on what those allergens might be, should be the first steps when diagnosing someone with inflammatory bowel disease. I think this is especially important if the person is diagnosed with Crohn's, Colitis or an autoimmune disease in general. If you have Crohn's disease or other intestinal disease and keep eating foods that you are sensitive to, you are only hurting your body and making your disease more difficult to manage. By eating foods that your body is reacting negatively to daily, you are just adding more inflammation in your body and tasking the immune system even more. One could argue that maybe Crohn's is a result of hidden food allergies that go on undiagnosed for years until it's too late and the inflammation finally is too much for the body to handle. The process varies from person to person and some people can live with the disease for several years before major problems where other people's bodies get sicker faster. The food intolerance and inflammatory bowel disease link is just my theory based on what I personally went through and know how my body is reacting to various foods . I wish they would study this link of hidden food allergies and inflammatory bowel diseases more. After reading countless stories of people who have Crohn's also have celiac or otherwise gluten intolerance, one starts to wonder if there is a link. The question is, is Crohn's possibly the result of the celiac or gluten intolerance and other food sensitives or is Crohn's causing the food sensitivities? There is so much more we don't understand but more research needs to be done on the effects of the diets, food allergies and inflammatory bowel diseases.

If you suspect you have issues with foods or you've never had food allergy testing done, I encourage you to do it. It was the first step that helped me to get to the root of why my body was reacting the way it was. You can order the stool test by yourself like I did. I just used Enterolabs for the test and ordered it online on my own. They sent me the stool test kit with instructions on how to do everything and how to return it. There are other companies as well that can do the testing for you so I encourage you to do some research and just pick the company that feels right to you.

Root Causes and Modern Medicine

My doctor tried to give me another prescription of Asacol and I refused. I told him I didn't need it because I was feeling better than I ever had and I had no pains or other symptoms. I tried telling him about my diet but he wasn't listening. He wrote in my chart "patient refuses treatment". I told him he could write whatever he wanted. I left and never went back. This was several years ago. All this led me to start learning even more about diets and the root causes of autoimmune diseases. I was determined to figure out how to help my body. For the first time in so many years I was feeling amazing. I didn't have the constant runs to the bathroom and my daily pains had disappeared. I learned more about functional medicine and how autoimmune disease work by doing countless of hours of research online. Functional Medicine vs Modern Medicine

The unfortunate fact is that today's modern medicine is reactive to medical situations and is not interested in getting to the root causes of the diseases or about the prevention for that matter. The conventional medicine is more of the Band-Aid approach to diseases with waiting until your body breaks down and then managing it with prescription drugs. The medicines don't really cure the disease but mask the symptoms, which is especially the case with medicines made for autoimmune diseases. Many of those medicines are immune suppressants meaning, they shut down your immune system which stops your immune system from attacking itself but it doesn't address what is causing your immune system to be on an overdrive to begin with. When your immune system is suppressed with the medicines, you open the body to possibilities of other diseases, including cancer. A dear friend of mined died from Colitis and cancer brought on by her medicines several years ago. I wish I could have helped her but at the time I didn't know as much as I know now. Once you figure out what is triggering your immune system to not function correctly, such as food allergies or leaky gut, you can start the healing process by removing that trigger. This is how functional medicine doctors approach medicine. They look for the root cause of why the body is not healthy and why the body is showing signs of illness. Functional medicine also believes that diseases start in the gut so addressing your gut health is the first thing they do. It wasn't until I understood this concept that I was able to help my own body and gut to heal, and as a result started feeling better than I had in years.

Leaky Gut and skin issues

Leaky gut is one of the leading causes for autoimmune diseases as well as skin related issues such as psoriasis, eczema etc. I personally have psoriasis on top of having Crohn's disease and I was able to get rid of my psoriasis by addressing my gut health and healing it.

Leaky gut is something that many people have without even knowing it. It can manifest itself in many different ways including mental issues such as depression, sadness, overwhelm, brain fog, skin issues, frequent colds, etc. Gut health has a direct link to the brain and many medical conditions as well. When I removed gluten from my diet, my brain fog disappeared and so did my psoriasis. I didn't really even realize I had brain fog, until it was gone. The clarity I gained in the way my brain and mind worked was incredible. Had I not experienced it myself, I wouldn't have believed the difference. I didn't even understand I had a problem until the problem was gone. I felt better than I had in years. I had gotten used to not really ever feeling that good; having headaches and brain fog thinking it was normal part of life. When all of it disappeared it was an amazing feeling. My brain fog is still gone today and I very rarely get headaches.

What is a leaky gut?

Basically leaky gut means that the proteins from food get through your intestinal walls undigested, causing hosts of problems in your body. Your body doesn't recognize the proteins in the blood and mistakenly identifies them as a threat causing the body to start attacking itself, hence autoimmune response.

In order help your body do what it's designed to do naturally, it's imperative to pay attention to your gut health and help your gut heal if you are suffering from leaky gut or other gut issues such as imbalance of good bacteria. Every time you take a course of antibiotics you kill off the good bacteria from your gut along with the bad. If you don't work on replacing the gut with the good bacteria again you leave it vulnerable to future problems. Ways to add healthy bacteria into your gut is with probiotics, kefir, yoghurt (only high quality no processed and sugar filled yoghurts with junky ingredients), fermented foods (sauerkraut etc.). If you can't tolerate dairy, goat milk yogurts are great. Almond milk and coconut milk yogurts can be beneficial too but keep an eye on the ingredients and try to choose yogurts without additives and fillers such as gums which can cause additional stomach issues.

How do you heal a leaky gut?

Probiotics are extremely important part of the diet for anyone suffering with intestinal disorders or autoimmune diseases. The bacteria balance in your gut affects your health, digestive process and your body's ability to defend against diseases. Your gut health also can be linked with food sensitivities. There are some things besides taking probiotics that can help heal the lining of the gut. Bone broth and bone broth protein powder has been found to be beneficial. Collagen and gelatin has been found to help the body as well. One of my favorite books on this subject is Dr. Axe's Eat Dirt. I highly recommend you read it to learn more about the importance of gut health and the link with your overall health. I personally make sure I get probiotics from food everyday either in a supplement or by eating high quality organic, plain yoghurt. I also eat bone broth protein daily because I'm not a fan of bone broth by itself. I also stick to a very clean diet and avoid junky ingredients that negatively affect your gut health such as high fructose corn syrup, hydrogenated oils and processed vegetable oils such as canola and soybean oil.

What finally put me on the path of healing & My Diet

In my personal case my biggest trigger for my Crohn's disease and the symptoms ended up being undiagnosed gluten allergy and several other food sensitives that I was able to eliminate with a long gut healing process, except the gluten intolerance. The reason I know this for sure is because of the testing I had done that revealed the sensitives. Also every time I've tried to eat gluten, my Crohn's symptoms come back. As long as I stay on my diet and stay 100% gluten free, my Crohn's stays in remission and I don't have the typical symptoms of pains, fullness, constant bathroom runs etc. I have also been medication free ever since which is several years now. If I get an occasional stomach upset form eating out despite eating gluten free, I use essential oils to help my stomach.

After many years on the Paleo diet and a regimen of supplements etc., I started slowing adding foods that were not allowed on traditional Paleo diet such as organic, full fat dairy, corn (I missed Mexican food like crazy), beans, lentils, potatoes etc. I introduce them one by one and noticed that I didn't get a reaction. I did try to introduce gluten and that didn't go over very well. My Crohn's symptoms returned instantly. I tried a few times again a few years later and I realized I couldn't have gluten without feeling horrible. Gluten in food causes my body to react and my Crohn's symptoms (pains, cramping, having to run to the bathroom) come   back   instantly.

What's a Paleo Diet?

It's a diet based on the types of foods presumed to have been eaten by early humans, consisting of meat, fish, vegetables, and fruit, and excluding dairy or grain products and processed food.

Foods allowed on the paleo diet

- Grass-fed meat
- Fish/seafood
- Eggs
- Fresh fruits and vegetables
- Nuts and seeds (except peanuts, peanuts are considered legumes which are not allowed)
- Olive oil and other healthy fats such as coconut oil, grassfed butter, avocado oil

What foods are not allowed on Paleo diet?

- All processed foods
- Cereal
- All Grains (corn, wheat, oats etc)
- Legumes (beans, lentils etc including peanuts)
- Refined Sugar
- Potatoes
- Refined vegetable oils (canola oil, soybean oil etc)
- Dairy

What can you do to support your body with starting a healing process?

If getting allergy testing done is not possible for you right away and you want to know the things you can try now, here are some things that I would suggest for you.

These may or may not help you since everyone's body is different and the gut microbe is different but it's worth the try. These are things that I've learned over the years and have helped me. I also follow these guidelines personally to manage my disease.

If you do get food allergy testing done, I highly recommend a stool test because blood tests are not found to be as accurate. I personally had a stool test done years ago that revealed the foods that I was allergic to at the time. Today I can eat 2 out of the 3 foods that I was allergic to per the test results. This is because after going on the healing journey focusing on making my gut healthier, I can now eat those foods that previously caused me problems.

If you have Crohn's, Colitis or IBS and you are reading this, I urge you to go 100% gluten free. Not partial but 100%. You can't go partially gluten free because it won't allow your body to heal and get the allergen out of your body. Also please note that wheat (gluten) today is not the same wheat your grandparents ate several years ago. The wheat harvested and used in breads today is a lot higher in gluten content than wheat used to have. It's also sprayed with pesticides especially Roundup which is linked to several health problems with the recent headlines of Roundup causing cancer. The reason so many people have gluten allergy now is partly because the modern wheat is extremely hard for the body to digest having a higher gluten content and many people have leaky gut or bacteria imbalance in the gut. In the olden days bread was made with sourdough dough where the bacteria actually helped to breakdown the gluten in the bread allowing your body to digest the bread easier. Also the wheat grown years ago, had a lower gluten level. Today's wheat is higher in gluten content and most bread sold and eaten today is not sourdough and even if it is sourdough bread, it has not been produced with the same way it used to be produced. True sourdough bread takes several days to produce because the dough has to ferment and the fermentation process is what helps to breakdown some of the gluten in.

Today's commercial sourdough bread is made completely differently with quick rising yeast etc. There are some true artisan breads available still but those are very hard to find and you certainly won't find them in your grocery store. The "artisan" bread sold in grocery stores is not the real artisan bread produced with healthier wheat and baking process as the real sourdough bread despite what the label says. There are some smaller bakeries that you might be able to find real artisan bread from not made with the modern wheat or with the modern processes. Look for small bakeries at farmer's markets or online. I personally can't have even the real artisan sourdough breads (I've tried a few times) because my body doesn't do well with any gluten whatsoever so I just completely stay away. Everyone's body is different though so it's best to try and find what works for your body.

Dairy can also give problems so going dairy free can be beneficial, at least for short term. If you choose dairy, be sure to choose organic options.

How to Get Started With Healthier Diet

Getting started with a healthier lifestyle and diet is super simple. It might sound intimidating but I'm here to break it down for you in easy steps. There is no magic to it. It's just about eating real foods and keeping away from processed foods as much as possible.

Throw out all processed foods from your pantry. Only eat foods that come from the nature, foods that have not been processed or manufactured in factory with a long list of ingredients. Eat fruits, vegetables, coconut oil, grassfed butter, grassfed meat, fish, chicken preferably organic, eggs, nuts (no peanuts) and seeds. If your stomach is not handling food very well, start with healthy smoothies with organic frozen foods, coconut or almond milk and high quality protein powder preferably grassfed or bone broth and almond butter. Add collagen or bone broth protein if using regular protein powder. Only choose organic dairy products or if dairy is bothering you or you are following a paleo diet, choose almond milk or coconut milk. Add fish oil supplements, digestive enzymes, bone broth protein powder, collagen and vitamin D3 supplements (see the resources section for suggested supplements and where to buy them). Also take a high quality probiotic supplement or consume fermented foods such as sauerkraut and kefir daily. Also have yoghurts without junky ingredients. Only choose organic, full fat yogurts or almond milk or coconut milk yoghurts if you can't tolerate dairy or you are following a paleo diet. Goat's milk yogurts are an excellent option as well. Also add a healthy wholefoods based vitamin supplement. Be sure to check with your doctor if using or adding any supplements to your diet, especially if you have existing medical concerns and/or you are taking medication. If you can tolerate dairy be sure to choose organic and preferably grassfed dairy products.

Sample daily meals

Breakfast

A smoothie made with almond or coconut milk or organic milk if you can tolerate, frozen organic fruit, bone broth protein powder or collagen powder and grassfed protein powder, add greens (spinach or kale etc) if you can tolerate. Be cautious with green powders as they can have chlorophyll which can give more stomach problems especially if your intestines are already flaring. Add a probiotic powder or kefir for probiotics or eat yoghurt. If you eat yoghurt please be sure to avoid processed yogurts including Greek yogurt which are not healthy despite the advertising. Anytime the yoghurt is more processed with thickeners etc it becomes an unhealthy option. Choose goat milk yoghurts if you can't tolerate dairy or choose organic, grass-fed plain yoghurts and add your own gluten/grain free granola and fruit. Almond and coconut milk yoghurts can be ok too but watch for junky ingredients such as fillers and gums which can upset the gastrointestinal tract more. Instead of a smoothie you can also do organic eggs and bacon or breakfast sausage and some fruit Paleo diet style.

Lunch

Homemade salad with salad greens, vegetables (tomatoes etc), protein (such as organic eggs, nitrate free lunch meat, cooked chicken, smoked salmon etc) Drizzle with extra virgin olive oil and add some vinegar or already made salad from the store (verify no chemicals or additives are listed on the label). You can also make your own salad dressing or buy higher quality salad dressings without chemicals and additives. Just read the labels and verify that it only contains olive oil, vinegar and spices no high fructose corn syrup, canola oil etc.

Snack

Green tea Nuts and fruit or organic apple with almond
butter
Raw or organic cheese (if you can tolerate) and
fruit/vegetables or Larabar or Perfect Bars.
Paleo snack bars also work. Keep an eye on the ingredients
and double check the ingredients so that there are no
processed ingredients or additives (if you don't recognize the
ingredients as food, it's safe to say it's not something you
want to be eating). I personally like Larabars and Perfect bars
because they have healthy ingredients.

Dinner

Organic chicken or wild fish with cooked organic vegetables.
If you are craving pasta, have your favorite pasta sauce
without gluten and add zucchini or carrot noodles in lieu of
regular pasta. If you can tolerate gluten free pasta, then you
can use that. I personally eat my favorite pasta meals but I
just make them with gluten free pasta options available at
Trader Joe's and Target. When I was following a strict paleo
diet, I didn't use any grains including gluten free pastas.
Check paleo cookbooks and blogs for healthy options for
main meals. Avoid drinking a lot with meals if you have
digestion issues. Be sure to drink plenty of water though
throughout the day and avoid drinks with empty calories or
artificial sweeteners.

My Diet today

My Modified Paleo Diet

Today I follow my version of the paleo diet and have followed this diet for several years now. I continue to keep my disease in remission and I'm medication free. How I eat might not work for everyone but I want to share with you what I did to help my body so that you have a starting point on how to incorporate a healthier diet for yourself and see how that can affect your body. Everyone's body is different and reacts differently to food and diets but I encourage you to try different things.

Keep trying; keep searching until you find the answers and the right diet for you. Unfortunately doctors are not really trained on diets and the possibilities on diet and disease connections. Diets in general have a huge effect on our health so I can't imagine someone having an autoimmune disease and be told you can eat whatever you want. Doctors should be ordering food allergy tests automatically especially if you are dealing with Crohn's or Colitis or any autoimmune disease. Many times the underlying cause is a undiagnosed food allergy which can be stemming from a leaky gut. The unfortunate fact is that doctors don't look for the allergies.

Paleo diet is great one to try because it's really a diet just based on real foods, foods that your body can recognize as being food.

Eating packaged and processed foods puts a huge burden on your body because it has to deal with all those additives and chemicals added to the food and deal with the lack of nutrients. Also the junk foods hinder the gut microbiome and don't allow the good bacteria to thrive.

Keto is a very popular diet current. It's just a modern version of Atkins diet focused on high protein and fat consumption. I personally don't recommend keto especially if your gut is very badly inflamed because the extra protein and fat will be very hard on your body to digest. I recommend going on a Paleo diet instead. It's more sustainable in the long run and isn't focused on so much fats and protein as the keto diet is.

Keto diet is great to try short term for people who don't have gut related issues but I don't recommend it if your gut is very bad inflamed and you are not able to eat many foods to begin with.

When I initially went on the Paleo diet myself, it took me a long time to go through the healing process. There is no way my body could have handled the extra fat and protein required in Keto. As weak as I was from having to go to the bathroom so much, it would have been a disaster to go on ketosis, as is the goal with eating Keto diet, which means that your body burns fat instead of carbs for fuel. In order to get your body to make the switch you have to get to ketosis by limiting your carbs and mostly getting your calories from fat and protein. Trying to make a body to do if you already have very badly inflamed gut is very difficult for your body to handle so I definitely don't recommend it. I would do a Paleo diet instead and slowly start the healing process. If you want to try Keto once your body is feeling better, then that's different. I tried Atkins type diet years ago before I went on my healing journey and discovered Paleo and it personally made me feel horrible. I couldn't continue more than a day. My gut wasn't having it and I just felt horrible. When I went on the Paleo diet I never felt like that. I actually felt great and as the months went by I felt better and better.

Several years ago I slowly started adding foods not allowed on Paleo diet, such as potatoes, rice and corn to see how my body would react. I added the foods one by one and waited a few weeks to see if I had a reaction. My body seemed to handle the foods well except wheat (gluten). I tried to eat gluten foods on a few different occasion and my symptoms always returned. For this reason, I don't ever eat gluten. I strive to eat whole foods as much as possible and I stay away from processed foods with exception of occasional gluten free chips.

Here is what my diet consists of today: organic, full fat dairy preferably grass-fed, fruits and vegetables, organic eggs, organic rice, organic beans, lentils, grassfed meat, organic chicken, wild salmon, fish, occasional Mexican food (no wheat tortillas or wheat based sauces) seafood, wholefood based vitamin supplements including omega 3 and probiotics. I also use essential oils daily to support my body and the immune system as well as support my mood/stress level.

My sample daily diet

Breakfast

Organic, whole milk plain yoghurt with gluten or grain free granola and some fruit or eggs with a slice of gluten free toast or gluten free oatmeal with grassfed butter doTERRA Lifelong Vitality Supplements and DDR prime cellular support essential oil blend with a few drops of doTERRA lemon essential oil in the water. Please do not attempt to consume essential oils unless the bottle specifically states intended for internal usage. doTERRA is the only brand of essential oils I trust for internal usage and have used them personally for several years now. There are some precautions to follow if you are consuming essential oils, especially if you are taking medication or you are pregnant or breastfeeding. As a certified essential oil coach, I educate my clients on proper and safe usage of essential oils.

Lunch

Homemade salad made with tuna in olive oil or nitrate free lunch meat and a hard boiled organic egg drizzled with extra virgin olive oil and splash of vinegar. I don't use readymade salad dressing because of possible chemicals or ingredients that don't agree with my stomach such as xanthan gum or other gums which are fillers and binding agents used in processed foods.

Snack in the afternoon

Nuts and/or dried fruit or Larabar Green tea

Dinner

Organic chicken or fish, vegetables (either steamed or roasted). Sometimes I'll eat a paleo breakfast for dinner with organic eggs and grassfed beef, nitrate free hot dogs or bacon. I balance out my eating over a span of a few days or a week, and try to follow what my body craves. Some nights I crave a vegetarian meal so I eat it and sometimes I grave meat or fish. I try to tune into my body as much as possible and eat the healthy foods that I'm craving. By eating foods that I crave, I'm not talking about unhealthy foods such as French fries or hamburgers (wrapped in lettuce or with a gluten free bun) or chips. I do eat those kinds of "junk" foods occasionally but sparingly.

Night time

A cup of tea or coffee with organic cream or milk and a two squares of dark chocolate or other "healthier" sweets I never count calories. I just focus on eating whole foods and listening to my body. If I'm craving a certain food I'll eat it because I figure my body must need it. I don't mean eating junk foods but foods that are healthy that I might feel like eating that day.

Emotional Health

I take time every day to appreciate the small things and just be still for a moment. I do a daily gratitude journaling. I use essential oils to help reduce stress and help me manage emotions and moods as well as for supporting my immune system. Stress can really aggravate my Crohn's which is typical for autoimmune diseases. Stress is not good if you have any disease, especially an autoimmune one. I personally try to be mindful of the negative effects stress has on the body and I try to avoid it and control it as much as I can. It's not always easy running two businesses full time and being a mom and a wife running a household also but I try and do the best I can. I'm a certified Health and essential oil coach through American Association of Drugless Practitioners and doTERRA Wellness Advocate as well as a jewelry designer so my businesses keep me busy. I also try and take a few minutes and do self-care every day in the form of exercise, reading, walking etc., using essential oils and doing things I really love to do.

Remove Toxins

Removing toxins from your environment and personal care is important as well if you have autoimmune diseases because the chemicals just add to the load of your body having to process them. Not even mentioning the health consequences of toxins and chemicals in your body. I personally only use non-toxic cleaning products and laundry soap in our home. I also choose non-toxic body and skin care products as much as possible but I'm not entirely obsessed with it. I do use some mainstream makeup products for example but I strive to choose natural products when it comes to the skin since the skin is your biggest organ.

Resources

Some links might include affiliate links or are links to products I sell personally as a doTERRA Wellness Advocate. I'm sharing these resources because I personally use and trust these products and brands mentioned in the resources. These products have had a profound effect on my health, which is the reason I'm sharing them with others. I use these products daily myself and have for several years now.

My contact info

My Health & Essential Oil Coaching website www.reijaeden.com

My handmade jewelry line, including essential oil bracelets and necklaces www.redenjewelry.com

Supplements & Protein Powder

Bone brother protein powder by Dr. Axe - https://store.draxe.com/

Collagen or bone broth collagen by Dr. Axe - https://store.draxe.com/

Lifelong vitality Supplements by doTERRA (these have literally changed the way I feel every day and I have so much for energy. My previous hair loss stopped when I started using these and my hair started growing back. I have more energy than ever and I've never felt better.) - www.mydoterra.com/reijaeden

doTERRA Digestzen essential oil blend for occasional stomach upset - http://bit.ly/2KMh7BM

Digestive Enzymes by doTERRA – www.mydoterra.com/reijaeden

Coconut oil supplements if you don't like cooking or eating with coconut oil. Try and find organic options. Amazon is a great place to find them.

Probiotics – PB Assist + or PB assist Jr if using them for kids by doTERRA www.mydoterra.com/reijaeden

Non-toxic household cleaning products

The Honest Company
Seventh Generation
doTERRA Onguard line www.mydoterra.com/reijaeden
doTERRA Baby line www.mydoterra.com/reijaeden

Blogs

www.againstallgrain.com
www.elanaspantry.com
www.marksdailyapple.com
www.draxe.com
www.reijaeden.com

Books

Danielle Walker's Against All Grain cookbooks
Elana's Pantry Almond flour cookbooks
The Primal Blueprint
NomNom Paleo
Nourishing Traditions
Celeste's Best Allergen free cookbook
Eat Like a Dinosaur (paleo cookbook for kids)
Everyday Paleo
The Grain Free Family Table
Well Fed
Eat Dirt by Dr. Axe
Gather

www.ingramcontent.com/pod-product-compliance
Lightning Source LLC
Chambersburg PA
CBHW051401250726
48656CB00006B/2210